High Blood Pressure

Know the Causes, Signs, Symptoms and Treatment.

By Sally Pederson

Thank you for purchasing this book. Please review this
book on Amazon. I need your feedback so I can make
the next version even better. Thank you very much.

For other books by this author go to:
https://www.amazon.com/author/sallypederson

Introduction

Have you ever wondered how our heart pumps blood so that this life giving fluid is available to even the far-reaching corners of our body? Indeed, it is a classic example of pressure wherein our heart is naturally designed to apply the principle in a manner that effectively ensures that no organ is deprived of blood. Commonly referred to as blood pressure, it is essentially the force with which blood travels to and from the heart via various pipelines known as arteries and veins.

Nature's way of ensuring good health of any individual entails maintaining the blood pressure at a certain level that is ideally suited for performance of all bodily functions. But unfortunately this level cannot always be maintained since it is affected by a number of different factors and the outcome is its rise and fall, the former being high blood pressure and the latter being low blood pressure. Because both conditions are adverse for the well being of the individual, efforts must be made to keep them at bay and maintain normal blood pressure for as long as possible.

How is the change in blood pressure detected? There are various machines that enable an individual to measure his blood pressure and although these are readily available in the physician's clinic, keeping one at home is strongly recommended. If a particular person is susceptible to fluctuations in blood pressure then keeping a machine at home and learning how to operate it is sure to work in his favor. However, the decision as to which machine should be bought should be made only after conducting sufficient amount of research on the subject and carefully weighing the pros and cons of each.

In case the systolic and diastolic readings are found to have exceeded their mark, it is time for the individual to undertake corrective measures immediately in order to restore them to their normal levels. Prior to embarking on corrective action it is first imperative to identify the root cause so that an appropriate treatment method can be employed. There could be a number of underlying causes for high blood pressure and some of the common factors are obesity, sedentary lifestyle, poor eating habits, stress, smoking and alcohol.

Having adopted lifestyle changes, it would be unfair to expect immediate results. Given the fact that the blood pressure might have taken years to spin out of control, it is only logical that it will take some time to revert to its normal state. Under the circumstances, persistence and patience on part of the patient is the key to healthier and better living. Some of the pointers that should be adhered to are inclusion of fruits and vegetables in the diet while keeping salt content to the minimum, exercising regularly and learning relaxation techniques.

Blood pressure is not limited to a particular age group, ethnicity or gender and even though African Americans have been found to be more prone to it than others, this condition has been known to exist in children as well. Medications are of course there but trying to cure it in a natural way is something that is likely to reap long term benefits to patients. After all, we all have one body and one life and hence should take care of it in the best way possible.

Table of Contents –

HIGH BP AND RELATED HEALTH PROBLEMS

The force of blood against the walls of the artery is known as blood pressure. When blood pressure is measured, the reading is expressed by two numbers, one above and one below. While the number above indicates the force of blood on the arteries during heart-beats and is known as systolic pressure, the number below indicates the force of blood on the arteries in-between the beats and is known as diastolic pressure.

When blood pressure is normal, the reading would be 120/80 or even lower. If pressure is high, the reading would be140/90 or even higher. This is a condition known as hypertension or high blood pressure. Physical inactivity, stress, diet, medical conditions and medication, usage of tobacco, and alcohol, age and even ethnicity is shown to lead to and or have an impact on high blood pressure. Blood pressure higher than normal can put a person's life in jeopardy. Some of the health problems associated with high blood pressure are enumerated as follows -

Blurred or impaired vision – This occurs due to the bursting of blood vessels in the eyes.

Stroke - Due to either hardening of arteries in the brain in turn blocking the blood flow to the brain or thinning of the blood vessels in the brain causing them to balloon or burst, the victim suffers from stroke.

Kidney disease – It is caused when the blood vessels leading to the kidney are damaged. Effective removal of fluid and waste material is hindered, leading to the accumulation of more fluid in body, raising the blood pressure even more.

Heart attacks – As with the brain, the blood vessels surrounding the heart may be narrowed due to high blood pressure. This limits blood flow to the heart, reduces the amount of oxygen reaching the heart, causing chest pain. The complete blocking of the blood flow and the reduction of oxygen causes heart attack.

Congestive heart failure – With high blood pressure the heart is forced to pump blood against higher pressure which weakens the heart over time. This reduces the blood supply to other organs and leads to heart failure.

High blood pressure is a condition that anyone even children can develop. It is more common amongst the African-American segment, but life style also plays a main role in its development. Therefore what can be done to reduce high blood pressure?

Since obesity or being overweight increases the risk of developing high blood pressure and puts a person at higher risk of developing a heart disease, stroke or kidney failure, losing weight is imperative for causing a significant reduction of blood pressure. Increasing the intake of fresh fruits and vegetables and limiting the amount of salt in the diet reduces the risk of developing high blood pressure and also helps control it.

In addition, people with high blood pressure should have their blood pressure checked regularly. This can be done with a physician or at home. Since life style change alone would not help, patients of high blood pressure should consult a physician and get on medications that would help reduce their blood pressure.

Keeping a watch on blood pressure usually translates into a healthy life.

CREATING AWARENESS

Approximately 72 million people in the United States, twenty years and older suffer from high blood pressure. 28% are completely unaware that they are victims. Therefore if you are diagnosed with it, you are not alone.

According to statistics one in three adult Americans suffers from it. It is more common in young African-Americans than in the young white Americans. There are still huge percentages of people that are unaware of it. Therefore if someone feels that he or she is singled out, they should not feel that way.

Some people think that they are invincible. They like to believe that high blood pressure will never affect them and so never get their blood pressure checked. Chances are that they may have it and will never know, thus ending up with life threatening conditions. There are several ways of minimizing the risk of contracting high blood pressure and these methods also help alleviating and bringing it under control in victims already suffering from it. Exercise and life style changes are a great way of controlling high blood pressure.

The best way to start is by striving to reduce weight if overweight. Watching the pounds is important because people who are overweight easily develop high blood pressure. How do you lose this excess weight? Indeed, the best way is to start exercising. Exercise is a great method to lower blood pressure whether over weight or not. Also eating right is essential when it comes to losing weight.

Incorporating more fresh fruits and vegetables and reducing salt in the diet not only reduces blood pressure but is also a proven method of losing weight.

Reducing the amount of alcohol consumed is also important in decreasing blood pressure. If a person is a heavy smoker it would be a good idea to lessen the intake and gradually quit altogether. There are over-the-counter medication available to help quit and also counselors who could help in quitting. Stress is a common occurrence nowadays. If a person is burdened with a high amount of stress, techniques in relaxation should be practiced, for example, meditation or listening to music. It is entirely up to the person to decide which technique that improves the condition best.

A few interesting facts worth noting is that 90-95% of the time the causes for high blood pressure is unknown and that people with less levels of education and low income suffer more from high blood pressure. The latter may be due to high levels of stress prevalent amongst this section of the population. Easy detection methods and methods of control helps to reduce the risks associated.

Who develops high blood pressure is not really the heart of the matter - it is controlling the pressure from spinning out of control that matters the most. Seeing a physician, taking medication with life style change, making decisions together with a physician in finding the best method suited to finding methods of prevention, treatment and control are some of the measures that have proven to be effective in controlling blood pressure.

THE DEVELOPMENT HIGH BLOOD PRESSURE

A person may wonder why he or she developed high blood pressure. It is of no use wondering why. Methods of lowering it or controlling it should be sought, after having been diagnosed with it. Keeping a watch from the beginning is the best method of preventing the development of the condition. The fact that most people are unaware of the root cause of it is why people develop this condition in the first place. Though older age is the most common time to show signs of high blood pressure, it is better to start young in keeping it in check, thus lowering its probability of occurrence. To this effect, there are a few factors that need watching.

Obesity or weighing more than one should is a risk associated with high blood pressure. Reduction of weight, even if it is just ten pounds, can keep a dramatic check on blood pressure. Therefore, the onus is on the patient to never feel depressed for being overweight and living in the high risk category.

Maintaining a healthy diet is also a great way to losing weight. Keep a check on salt and sodium levels, as these have a negative effect on normal blood pressure levels. Limit the usage of salt and try finding a substitute that suits your palette. Increasing the amount of fruits and vegetables in the diet will not only reduce blood pressure but makes a person feel better as well. Tobacco and alcohol have shown to increase blood pressure. First and foremost reducing the consumption of these will reduce blood pressure levels to a certain extent.

Once reduced, try quitting altogether. This will help improve blood pressure levels even more.

Indulging in regular exercise regime aids in reducing the blood pressure. This may come as good news to those regular gym freaks, but may be bad news to the couch potatoes. In order to maintain optimum blood pressure levels, exercising for at least thirty minutes a day is a must. These thirty minutes may be spaced out to ten minute time slots for those who cannot spare thirty minutes in one go. Stress is also a major factor that elevates blood pressure levels. It is very common these days especially amongst young people. The best method to overcome stress is to find methods that aid in relaxation, such as meditation, listening to music or getting involved in a hobby.

High blood pressure can be a side effect due to a certain medication that is taken. It is best to consult a physician and discuss about the medication and stop it altogether if necessary. Ethnicity can also be a cause. High blood pressure is more common in African-Americans who develop it at an early age. They also have a high mortality rate due to stroke and kidney disease. However early detection can prove its worth.

Monitor blood pressure regularly and take precautions to control it with either life style change or medication or a combination of both. Talk to your doctor. Strive for better health today instead of putting it off for tomorrow.

FACTORS ASSOCIATED WITH HIGH BP

Quite a number of factors play a key role in increasing a person's blood pressure. These can be changed by simply changing one's life style. Blood pressure if not constantly kept in check may aggravate over the years without a person even realizing it. Therefore what are these factors that one should be cognizant of?

Obesity - If a person is overweight or obese there is a risk of developing high blood pressure. Consulting a doctor and striving to lose at least ten pounds makes a difference if at risk of high blood pressure or already living with high blood pressure.

Lack of physical activity or exercise - Exercising at least thirty minutes a day reduces blood pressure. Exercise does not have to be strenuous and the times can be spaced out to get a total of a thirty minute workout. Exercise also helps losing weight.

Diet - Eating healthy, i.e. less salt, more vegetables and fruit reduces blood pressure levels tremendously. Eating healthy will also aid in losing weight in case of being overweight.

Stress - Stress can break a person not only mentally but also physically. This could also lead to high blood pressure. Practicing relaxation techniques greatly helps in reducing stress.

Tobacco and alcohol - Higher the consumption of alcohol and tobacco, the greater is the risk of developing high blood pressure. Limiting the consumption or quitting completely should be considered. Talking to the physician and using prescribed or over the counter products could help getting rid of the habits.

Medical conditions - Sleeping disorders that disturb breathing while sleeping and also kidney diseases can cause high blood pressure. A person could get more awareness about it by talking to his or her physician.

Medication and drugs - It is best to consult a physician before taking certain medication and drugs as some may elevate blood pressure. Special attention has to be paid when considering oral contraceptives, anti-depressants, some medicines prescribed for the common cold, nasal decongestants, drugs for anorexia and steroids.

Apart from these factors which can be controlled there are others that cannot be controlled. One such factor is a person's ethnicity. An individual of African-American origin is at higher risk than any other ethnic group in developing high blood pressure. Another factor is age and people over fifty five come under the high risk category of developing high blood pressure. Family history also plays a role and although a person has no control over these factors, he or she certainly has control over his or her life style. A slight change in life style can certainly control the development of high blood pressure. Ultimately, the end results of high blood pressure may be devastating which is why efforts should be made to lead a life that is free from risk of high blood pressure.

MUST KNOW POINTS

Blood pressure could be described as the force of with which the blood pounds upon the walls of the arteries. Sudden elevation of this pressure in the arteries leads to high blood pressure or hypertension. Listed as follows are certain points to keep in mind if living with high blood pressure.

First understand the numbers. Blood pressure is read with two numbers. The one above is known as the systolic pressure and the one at the bottom is the diastolic pressure. The normal reading for blood pressure is 120/80. If the reading is 130/90, it means that a person is in hypertension stage which is like a warning sign of developing high blood pressure.

When blood pressure is constantly monitored, it can be decreased as required. If at all it was a sudden transition from normal to high, then the reason for this should be considered. This may be due to a change in the diet or reduction of exercise or even due to a new medication. Blood pressure could be monitored at home with ease. One point that needs to be specifically kept in mind is that regular consultation with the physician is imperative. By ensuring this, means of lowering blood pressure can be established and routinely observed to see which ones work and which ones do not click at all.

As specified above there are certain medications which cause the blood pressure to rise. Therefore a physician should be consulted if it is replaced by some other medication. This is important because increase in blood pressure can lead to strokes, heart attacks and kidney dysfunction. If a change in the diet has caused a rise in blood pressure the physician should be consulted. Increased salt intake and reduced intake of fresh fruits of and vegetables could be one of the reasons. Therefore limiting the intake of salt and incorporating fruits and vegetables in the diet can decrease the blood pressure.

Reduction or complete halt of exercise may also be a cause for high blood pressure. It is best to get going with exercise all over again. If the exercise was given up due to an accident or a fall which resulted in a fracture, which then resulted in high blood pressure, it is best to consult the physician and find a way around the problem. Limiting the intake of tobacco and alcohol helps alleviate high blood pressure. Many people are unaware that these can cause high blood pressure. Because reducing intake or quitting helps reduce high blood pressure, attention should be focused on resources that help quit these habits.

Taking medication according to the strength prescribed and making sure to take it without forgetting is essential. Forgetting medication may lead to disastrous results associated with high blood pressure such as stroke. Therefore it is best to device methods that will help a person remember, like leaving calendar reminders on a mobile phones or setting up alarms.

Constant monitoring, having a consultation with the physician, getting answers to all questions regarding high blood pressure, life style change and medication will help a person reduce high blood pressure and maintain a happy and healthy life.

CHILDREN AT RISK

Children and even babies are not out of risk developing high blood pressure. This is not as uncommon as many would think. Kidney or heart problems in babies lead to the development of high blood pressure while in case of older children the same could be attributed to factors like family history and obesity.

A child's diet has to be kept in check, together with regular monitoring of his or her blood pressure in order to minimize health risks. More and more children in this contemporary generation are obese courtesy of a sedentary life style and poor eating habits. Television, computers and games and programs associated with them have rendered children lazy and have discouraged them to venture outdoors. Thus, the onus is on parents to get children involved in outdoor activities in form of a sport in school or a nature walk which will benefit both parent and child.

Watching a child's diet is equally important. Train the child to eat healthy from the beginning. Limit the child's salt intake and reduce the amount of fast food the child eats. Fast food is also responsible for obesity in a child. Increase the amount of fresh fruits and vegetables by trying different recipes for vegetables, hoping that there will at least be one that the child will like. Family history of high blood pressure also puts a child at risk. Routine checkups will ensure if the child has the condition or not. If at all the child has high blood pressure, regular monitoring will help in its control.

Just like an adult a child too can undergo stress. They deal with it in ways different to adults. This can also lead to the increase in their blood pressure. Talking with a child is very important. This can help a parent or adult to find out what is going on in a child's mind and also help a child to deal with any problems, if any, in the correct manner without undergoing undue stress. Over all, it is important for the child to be happy.

If a teenager is into smoking or drinking it is best to talk about it. Alcohol and tobacco increases the risk of high blood pressure later on in life. Talking about it helps a child to understand the consequences and probably would convince him to opt out of it.

Where diet and exercise cannot control a child's blood pressure, medication will have to be prescribed. A physician will be able to prescribe medication along with a diet regime to help control the problem. It is worthwhile to keep in mind that blood pressure increases until a person is around fifty. It is therefore also worthwhile monitoring a child's blood pressure from an early age. This will aid in its control and also aid in minimizing the risks associated with it.

CONTROLLING HIGH BP IN YOUR CHILD

As a parent you may not be aware that your child is at a risk developing high blood pressure. It is not an uncommon event. Therefore it is up to a parent to help a child live a happy and healthy life by monitoring and regulating the child's blood pressure while he/she is still young.

If your child is obese he or she is at high risk developing high blood pressure. Each year more children are diagnosed as been obese according to researchers. This is because children are lacking in exercise thanks to modern technology. They are glued to the television or computers for hours on end, rather than running outside and playing. Eating fast food also increases the risk of obesity.

You as a parent should take control. Take them for walks, ride your bicycles, go swimming, do whatever outdoor activity that both of you enjoy. Exercising for thirty minutes with your child everyday will benefit both of you. This will also help the child stay active all his or her life. It is not necessary to stop the watching television or playing a game on the computer completely. Limiting this time is what is necessary.

Equally important is watching what your child eat. Start a diet regime for the whole family so that the child will not feel left out or bullied by older siblings. Make sure that the salt and sodium intake is reduced and a different seasoning is used instead. Introduce more vegetables and fresh fruits into the diet. This will ensure that the child will keep eating these even as an adult. Maintaining the specific daily dietary fiber requirement for a child is also very important. It should be as follows;

Children aged 01 - 03 years: 19 grams of fiber per day

Children aged 04 – 08 years: 25 grams of fiber per day

Female children aged 09 – 13 years: 26 grams of fiber per day

Male children aged 09 – 13 years: 31 grams of fiber per day.

Female children aged 14 – 18 years: 29 grams of fiber per day

Male children aged 14 – 18 years: 38 grams of fiber per day

As an adult you should consume 14 grams of fiber per thousand calories consumed. Nutrition labels should be consulted to make sure the daily dietary intake is been fulfilled. Make sure all meals are balanced as too much fat combined with physical inactivity would lead to obesity, in turn leading to high blood pressure. Send a balanced lunch for your child to have in school. Experiment with the menu until you have found one the child likes.

This does not mean that "junk food" should be completely ruled out. After all they are children. Choose a day during the week and a time where the whole family can enjoy some "junk food". Let the child be a child but with a healthier life style. You will both be thankful in the future. After all a healthy child means a happy parent.

MONITORING BP AT HOME

It is for the best that a person having high blood pressure should learn to monitor the same at home along with regular visits to the doctor. This constant monitoring will help decide if the changes in life style undertaken and medication have helped in reducing a person's blood pressure. It is best to keep a record of blood pressure when monitored at home as it will help decide what is working and what is not.

For monitoring blood pressure at home there are two types of monitors to choose from. One is the aneroid monitor, which uses a dial gauge with a pointer to aid reading the result. Aneroid monitors have a dial gauge and the blood pressure is read using a pointer. The cuff is inflated by hand, using a rubber bulb. The cuff also has an inbuilt stethoscope. These are portable and are cheaper than the digital monitors. However some people may find it difficult to inflate the cuff as the bulb is rather hard to squeeze and some find it difficult to hear as well.

On the other hand, with digital blood pressure monitors, the blood pressure is read using a screen. The cuff can either be manual or automatic. This also has an inbuilt stethoscope. As the screen shows numbers it is easy to read. Errors are reduced due to error codes and automatic deflation. There are monitors with an inbuilt paper printing facility, thus helping a person to keep a record of blood pressure readings. These are more expensive and as these are battery operated, the batteries have to be replaced every once in a while.

Finger or wrist monitors are also available, but these have proven to be inaccurate, more sensitive to movement and more costly. The correct cuff size is also important when considering the purchase of a blood pressure monitor as wrong cuff size has been known to lead to erroneous results.

When choosing a device it is best to choose one which has the correct cuff size to suite a person. If unsure, it is best to ask the physician. Always read the instructions and operate accordingly. Choosing one that is easy to read is essential. If it is confusing to operate, higher the chances are that the readings will be wrong.

Considering the amount a person is willing to spend on a monitor is also important. While making up your mind regarding purchasing one, someone who already uses one can be consulted. There are some brands that they may be able to recommend. These brands may be what they have used before or are still using. This would enable a person to decide which brand to purchase and which brand to avoid.

Even though blood pressure is monitored at home, a visit to the physician is essential. It is the physician after all who prescribes the medication. Constant monitoring and managing blood pressure reduces chances of stroke, kidney disease, heart attacks and helps leading a normal and healthy life.

A physician would be able to assist in correct usage of the monitor. Using it correctly will help a person benefit from the monitor purchased by him or her. Before monitoring blood pressure the following guidelines should be observed:

- ✓ Do not drink caffeinated drinks or alcohol or use products containing tobacco thirty minutes before taking a reading.
- ✓ Use the rest room.
- ✓ Relax
- ✓ Do not talk three to five minutes before taking the reading.
- ✓ Be comfortable. Keep back straight and refrain from crossing arms and legs.
- ✓ Make sure the arm is at the same level as the heart.
- ✓ Rest the arm on a table or hard surface.
- ✓ Fit the cuff snugly but make sure it yet has room for one finger to pass through.
- ✓ The cuff should be one inch away from the crease of the elbow.

Understand the reading. A reading of 120/80 or less is considered normal, while a reading of 160/100 or higher is considered high. A reading in-between these readings are considered as pre-hypertension, meaning that a person can develop high blood pressure in future. If the numbers are greater than normal it is best consulting a physician. With the aid of a physician the best possible way in controlling blood pressure could be discussed, like life style change, medication or a combination of both.

Few people are aware of the fact that one's blood pressure rises with age. Hence, when you monitor and take charge of your blood pressure early, you will be able to prolong your life span. The following are different ways to monitor one's blood pressure as also the advantages of doing the same -

Investing in a good device for monitoring blood pressure is great because it saves you the hassles of visiting the doctor's clinic every now and then. Those having high blood pressure should definitely go for this device. While young people may not really care about monitoring their blood pressure, but it is advisable to do so, especially if high blood pressure runs in one's family.

When keeping an eye on your blood pressure level, try to find out the reason behind its rise. This will be able to help you tackle the problem better. Following are some of the main culprits behind rise in blood pressure level:

Intake of tobacco and alcohol – The intake of alcohol and tobacco can dramatically increase one's blood pressure levels. In order to keep your blood pressure level at a safe level, try to abstain from consuming these two harmful items. You can take professional help in order to quit smoking or drinking completely.

Obesity – We all know that obesity is the primary cause of a lot of health problems, including rise in blood pressure. Losing weight is an extremely effective method of bringing down one's blood pressure level. Try reducing ten pounds and see what difference it makes.

Being physically inactive – If you just sit around the entire day and do not engage in any form of exercise then your blood pressure level is bound to rise. It is a well-known fact that working out regularly can keep the blood pressure level under check. It is recommended to engage in at least half an hour of physical activity on a daily basis. You do not have to go for thirty minutes of exercise at a stretch and can break it up into different sessions.

Stress – Another culprit behind high blood pressure levels is stress. Try de-stressing and relaxing yourself everyday through meditation to bring your blood pressure level down.

Diet – An unhealthy diet can cause the blood pressure to rise. Try to cut down on your salt consumption and include more fresh vegetables and fruits in your diet while reducing intake of fats.

Sleeping disorder – If there is an interruption in your breathing when you are sleeping then your blood pressure can rise. Seek doctor's help in case you have a sleeping disorder because medications can work wonders in treating such disorders.

Drugs from pharmacy stores – Certain drugs can cause blood pressure to rise like oral contraceptives, medicines for treating common cold, anti-depressants and nasal decongestants. Seek your doctor's advice regarding which medicines to avoid and which to consume.

By following the tips mentioned in this article, you will be able to keep your blood pressure level in check, thus reducing the odds of a kidney disease or a heart disease happening. Start now because it is never too late to take charge of your health.

What Do BP Numbers Mean?

Those who are worried about their blood pressure should fall into the practice of monitoring it from time to time in the comfort of their own home. Of course, it is still necessary to go for a blood pressure check-up from a doctor occasionally. In order to be able to monitor one's blood pressure, one should first find out the meaning of blood pressure numbers.

When it comes to blood pressure reading, there are two numbers – one is at the top and the other is at the bottom. While the one on top signifies the person's systolic pressure, the one at the bottom signifies his/her diastolic pressure. Diastolic pressure can be defined as the force of blood present in the arteries when the heart is relaxing between two beats while systolic pressure is the force when the heart is beating.

Blood pressure readings can be segregated into four groups or categories - normal blood pressure, pre-hypertension, stage 1 hypertension and stage 2 hypertension. The first one, i.e. normal or regular blood pressure is when the reading of systolic pressure is less than 120 while the diastolic pressure reading is under 80. It is read as 120/80 and those having this reading are leading a healthy life.

Pre-hypertension, which is the second category is when the systolic pressure reading is anywhere between 120-139 and the diastolic reading is anywhere between 80 and 89. The lowest pre-hypertension reading is 121/81 while the highest one is 139/89. In case your blood pressure reading is categorized as pre-hypertension then you should keep a close supervision on your lifestyle in order to prevent the blood pressure from rising.

Stage 1 hypertension, or the third category is when one's systolic pressure reads 140-159 and the diastolic pressure reads 90-99. The individuals whose blood pressure reading falls under this category adopt measures to lower their blood pressure. This can be done either through meditation or other methods suggested by the doctor.

The fourth category in blood pressure readings would be Stage 2 hypertension. Here, the systolic pressure would read 160 or higher and the diastolic pressure would read 100 or higher. Falling into this category is akin to being in the danger zone because it can lead to serious health complications. Thus, if your blood pressure reading falls into this category then you should engage in a lot of exercise and watch your weight closely. You might even need to resort to some medication.

At times one can fall into the Stage 2 hypertension because of the medicines one might be consuming, like nasal decongestants, anti-depressants, medicines for cold or oral contraceptives. In case you are worried about your blood pressure level then speak to a doctor. Take charge of your health to lead a better life, try to eat a healthy diet consisting of vegetables and fruits and avoid drinking or smoking. In case you have a pet dog then it would be a good idea to take it for walk everyday. By doing this, you will not only be able to improve your dog's health but also your own and have fun while you are at it.

POINTERS TO KEEP

Whether you already have high blood pressure or you want to avoid having high blood pressure, it is possible to do so without consuming any medication. Changes in lifestyle habits can trigger high blood pressure. However, the good news is that there is help for it. Now, all methods of reducing or controlling high blood pressure may work for you. At times, medications may also need to be administered side-by-side in order to lead a healthier life. Doctors are the best person to turn to in such a situation.

First things first, to control your blood pressure you should keep an eye on your weight. Try to reduce weight until you reach a healthy weight for your body. Obesity and high blood pressure go hand in hand, therefore to avoid this problem, reduce weight and watch what you eat. Many people are unsure about what their healthy weight is and if you are one of them then you can consult a doctor. Alternatively, you can use an online website in order to calculate your Body Mass Index or BMI, which is the ideal weight according to your height and age.

Controlling blood pressure can never be done without exercise or some sort of physical activity. Even if you do not like exercising, you have to engage in it in order to maintain a healthy blood pressure level. The rule of the thumb here is to exercise for thirty minutes every day, either at a stretch or by breaking down into several shorter sessions. Running and walking are particularly useful here.

Try to cut down on foods that are rich in salt or sodium from your diet. You can find out the recommended amount of sodium and salt from your physician or doctor and use herbs and spices instead of salt in order to flavor your food. When eating out, try to stick to your diet as closely and opt for the 'no salt' option whenever possible or at least ask for reduced amount of salt in your food. People generally consume more amounts of salt than they should but they are unaware of the same, which leads to health complications like high blood pressure.

Stress can be your number one nemesis when you are trying to reduce and maintain your blood pressure level. Different people prefer different methods of unwinding and de-stressing, so you should find something that works for you. Always practice meditation at the end of the day to get rid of all the stress and prepare your body for rest.

Changing your lifestyle habits and sticking to the new set of rituals also helps. You might want to note down the changes that you have made in your lifestyle so as to see whether it is effective for reducing blood pressure or not. In case these at-home tips do not help you then you might have to rely on professional intervention and opt for treatments. The doctor would be more than happy to enlighten you about the same so as to make you feel more at ease and less nervous.

PREVENTING HIGH BLOOD PRESSURE

In order to battle high blood pressure it is best first to start by making life style changes and at times life style changes prove to be so effective that medication is not necessary.

Try to quit smoking altogether. Smoking has a negative effect on blood pressure. It can increase it. Reduce alcohol to around two glasses a day and nothing more as this too tends to increase blood pressure. Exercising at least thirty minutes a day helps maintaining blood pressure levels at a normal range. If thirty minutes cannot be set aside in one go, consider spacing it out to ten minute intervals.

Eat healthy. Limit the intake of salt because salt increases blood pressure. Find an alternative seasoning to salt. There has to be one that you like. Increase the amount of fresh fruits and vegetables and steer clear away from fatty food. Obesity or being over weight is also harmful. Lose ten pounds at first and see the difference. You will see your pressure drop dramatically. This will motivate you to lose more.

Present day life style puts a person under undue stress. Undue stress increases blood pressure. Jobs, coping up with family life are examples of some stress related factors. Try avoiding stressful situations as much as possible. De-stressing methods such as medication is a great way of relieving stress.

There are certain factors that cannot be controlled which relate to high blood pressure. Ethnicity is one of them. African-Americans are at a greater risk than any other ethnic group. Age is another factor. If you are above fifty five consider yourself in the risk group. Family history is another. If any of these factors relate to you, you might need to start controlling diet, exercise regularly and reduce weight as means of precaution.

Certain medication such as nasal decongestants, drugs for anorexia, oral contraceptives, pain killers, antidepressants, cold medicines are also found to be culprits. The doctor that a person consults should always be aware of the medication he or she takes. Talk to your doctor about the precautionary methods and medications you can take to control blood pressure levels.

High blood pressure leads to stroke, heart attacks and kidney disease. It is best to talk to a doctor about the questions you may be having regarding high blood pressure. Get answers to all questions. No question is silly when considering your health. After all it is your life.

WATCHING WHAT YOU EAT

Even with a person who never had a problem of high blood pressure there could be a chance of developing it later on. Watching the diet from the beginning is a very good idea when talking about keeping high blood pressure in check.

A vegetarian diet could be tried where the following would be included - calcium, magnesium, vitamin A and C, potassium, complex carbohydrates, polyunsaturated fat and fiber. These have a great power in controlling blood pressure. Limiting the intake of sugar is beneficial. The common table sugar especially has shown to increase blood pressure. Foods which are high in fiber not only help reduce blood pressure but also prove effective in losing weight and reducing cholesterol.

Food that is low in fat, cholesterol and saturated food low blood pressure. Therefore a diet which include plenty of fruits, fresh vegetables, low fat dairy food, food less in cholesterol and saturated fat reduce blood pressure. The diet should also contain less salt. Salt directly affects blood pressure therefore should be kept at bay. A diet less in sodium and more in potassium reduces the effect of adrenaline this in turn reducing blood pressure. If sodium intake is reduced, potassium content should be increased.

Certain vegetables and spices also help in the control of blood pressure. There are some that a person that may not even be aware of. The essential oils in onions help and including two to three tables spoons a day help reducing the systolic blood pressure levels. Tomatoes are high in GABA, which helps lower blood pressure. Carrots and broccoli have compounds that reduce blood pressure. Increasing the amount of vegetables in a meal keeps blood pressure in check with or without having the problem of high blood pressure. Eating a clove of garlic a day is beneficial to the hearts. Celery is also a great vegetable to be added to the diet whenever possible.

It would be worthwhile to bear in mind that whatever food that is limited or increased is done for maintaining good health. The older a person gets healthier the food should be. Older people find that they enjoy healthier food. Any questions should be clarified with a doctor.

Health after all is wealth. Taking care of it will make a person definitely feel good about ones self.

METHODS OF LOWERING YOUR BP

Did you know that your diet, your habits, and the amount of exercise you get have an effect on your blood pressure? If you are living with high blood pressure or want to prevent getting high blood pressure there are certain things to be done in order to prevent or control it. Regular monitoring is necessary to ensure you have not contacted the disease or are maintaining the levels at the proper rate if suffering from it. Regular check ups with the doctor therefore is essential. Also there are different methods that could be employed to control it or preventing contacting it.

High blood pressure increases the risk of stroke, heart and kidney dysfunction along with damaging the blood vessels. Therefore getting the correct treatment is necessary. Life style changes help but may not show a dramatic improvement. For this medication has to be considered along with life style change.

Quitting tobacco is a way to reduce high blood pressure. Nicotine narrows blood vessels making the heart beat faster. This raises the heart beat increasing blood pressure. There are products available that would aid in quitting.

Eating healthy and exercising regularly also help lowering blood pressure. Obesity increases the risk of high blood pressure and makes it difficult to control. Planning a regime and adhering to it, together with recording the progress is a great way to know what suits a person, what works and what does not. Plenty of fresh fruit and vegetables, a low fat diet, less sodium and salt intake, reducing alcohol and caffeine intake is a good method of keeping blood pressure levels in check.

Stress is a common feature in the contemporary lifestyle of today and can affect blood pressure. Practicing techniques helps reducing stress. A doctor could also help in finding the best method to suit a person's need. If all these prove to be non-beneficial medication has to be sought. This may have to taken for the rest of a person's life. As this will help on the long run it should not be considered as a problem.

Read on the subject and talk to the doctor about any question you may have pertaining to high blood pressure. There is no question that is un-intelligent when it comes to health. These are essential for a person to live a long happy and more or less normal life.

METHODS TO CONTROL YOUR BP

Have you been diagnosed as having high blood pressure? Do you have a problem controlling it? In this article we will be discussing as to how you can take charge and control your blood pressure.

Age, ethnicity, family history and life style play a key role when talking about the development of high blood pressure. African-Americans are at a higher risk than any ethnic group in developing high blood pressure. A person who is above fifty five is more prone to develop it. Ethnicity, age or family history are factors which are non-controllable, but life style is a factor which is controllable.

Lower the intake of salt or sodium, the better it is for a blood pressure patient. A doctor can help you decide the levels you should be taking. Incorporate more fruits and vegetables. This will not only lower your blood pressure but will also help you feel better.

Start exercising. If physically inactive it can cause your blood pressure to increase. Thirty minutes a day is the recommended time limit for exercise. If this is not possible in one go, space the time out to five or ten minute intervals. Somehow manage to get the thirty minutes of exercise every day.

A person hooked on to smoking and drinking alcohol can have problems of high blood pressure. If so, reducing or quitting completely though tough, will work wonders. Try reducing initially, and slowly work your way to quitting. There are resources that can help a person quit. Find out about them and limit being around people who smoke and/or consume alcohol. Try doing something else if the need arises to smoke or drink.

If you are under a lot of stress due to your job or otherwise it is worth while noting that this could increase your blood pressure. Find a method that suits you to relax. It could be a hobby or meditation. This could be done as often as you like to keep undue stress at bay. Talking with your doctor also helps. Ask any question and get clarifications. A doctor can help with the best of methods to help you control your blood pressure. It might be essential to get on medication.

Take control and do the best for your health.

EXERCISE FOR CONTROLLING HIGH BP

What many people do not realize is that regular exercise can help control high blood pressure. It actually plays a key role in controlling the condition. The risk of developing high blood pressure increases as a person age. Age cannot be controlled but blood pressure can be controlled. High blood pressure leads to stroke, heart failure and kidney dysfunction. So why make yourself susceptible to the risk? Instead you must start controlling it now so that to enjoy many long years of good health.

Exercise strengthens the heart muscle. This causes the heart to pump blood easily reducing the pressure in the arteries. Exercise lessens the blood pressure at least by 10 millimeters. Exercising regularly benefits a person who may not be suffering from the condition by preventing its development during later stages of life. This also helps a person lose weight and maintain a desired weight. A person if overweight is more prone to developing high blood pressure.

Start exercising slowly at first and gradually increase the time and intensity. Find a regular routine more suited to you. Thirty minutes every day is sufficient enough but, as time plays a major factor in every ones lives, it can be spaced to ten minute intervals throughout the day if one cannot spare thirty minutes at a stretch. If a man is over forty and a woman over fifty it is best to talk to a doctor before starting an exercise regime. There are certain dos and don'ts when it comes to that age group. Smokers also have to consult the doctor, because smoking increases blood pressure and makes exercising difficult for a person.

Apart from having high blood pressure, having high levels of cholesterol and other underlying medical conditions have to be considered before exercising. Consult your doctor now and get diagnosed if unaware about other medical conditions before starting exercise. Strenuous exercise might be risky with other medical conditions. Be sure to warm up before exercising. Increase gradually after starting slowly. Breathe throughout without holding your breath, as holding your breath could cause blood pressure to increase and this is what we want controlling in the first place.

Keep a track of your progress of exercise. Monitor your blood pressure regularly to get to know your progress. If any pain or discomfort is felt during exercises notify the doctor immediately. Regular monitoring can be done by purchasing a home blood pressure monitor. Check your pressure before and after exercise. You have to know how much exercise is helping you.

Frequent exercise will help you lower your blood pressure levels if already high and prevent a person who does not have it from getting it. By this, chances of developing stroke, heart failure and kidney dysfunction is kept in check. Talk to your doctor as soon as possible and decide on a routine that will suit you. No matter how old you are and what ethnicity you are from, what your family history or gender is it is never too late to start exercising.

MEDICATIONS FOR HIGH BP

People who are diagnosed with high blood pressure change their lifestyle only to find that it does not have much effect. Lifestyle changes solely do not help and they need to be combined with specific medication for high blood pressure. Medications are generally used in combination, meaning two medications are used together. These are of many different types. The following medications are what is been used to treat high blood pressure -

- Alpha-Blockers decrease blood pressure by reducing nerve impulses to the blood vessels, allowing easy flowing.

- Alpha-Beta-Blockers have the same mechanism as Alpha-Blockers and in addition reduce the blood pumping through the vessels reducing blood pressure.

- Nervous System Inhibitors control the nerve impulses which relax the blood vessels. This widens the vessels and decreases the blood pressure.

- Beta-Blockers decrease the heart beat by reducing the nerve impulses to the heart and blood vessels, in turn reducing blood pressure.

- Diuretics, also known as "water pills", work on the kidney. These flush out the extra sodium and water.

- Vasodilators reduce blood pressure by the direct opening of the blood vessels. This is done by relaxing the muscles of the vessel walls.

- ACE Inhibitors namely Angiotensin converting enzyme, prevents the formation of the hormone angiotensin II, which causes the blood vessels to narrow. The medication relaxes blood vessels aiding in blood pressure decrease.

- Angiotensin Antagonists counter-act the action of angiotensin II on the blood vessels allowing them to widen and in turn the blood pressure is reduced.

- Calcium Channel Blockers prevent the entry of calcium in to the heart muscle cells and blood vessels causing the blood pressure to decrease.

Along with medication a few life style changes can make a difference, such as substituting salt for other seasoning, adding fresh fruits and vegetables and maintaining a healthy diet. Exercising everyday for thirty minutes can make a difference. The thirty minutes can be spaced into ten minute slots.

Keeping stress levels at check is as important. Involvement in a hobby, meditation is some methods that can help de-stress. It is best to try out a few methods and find one that works best. Cutting back or quitting alcohol and tobacco is a must when dealing with high blood pressure. This is not easy in one go but there are products available to help a person quit these habits.

Talking with the physician is beneficial. Regular visits and regular check ups will aid in coming up with the best medication and life style changes. Asking questions is equally important as doubts can be cleared. Also it is beneficial to tell the physician about other drugs been taken such as oral contraceptives and cold medication as these could also increase blood pressure.

REMEMBERING TO TAKE YOUR MEDICATION

Reminding one's self to take medication, especially if it is more than one at a time is a tedious task. Medication for high blood pressure is no exception. There are a few methods that could help a person remember to take the medication.

There are little pill boxes available that could help organize the pills a person has to take. These have one for every day of the week. All the pills that have to be taken for the day could be put in to each box. This is handy for anyone even if they don't forget. Try keeping medication on the bathroom sink. This will help a person remember to take the medication after brushing the teeth or after getting ready. This method is a simple way of reminding.

Taking the medication at the same time everyday is a good way of reminding one's self. It will then become a habit and will never be forgotten. If the medication has to be taken with food, take them with lunch. This has proven to be a useful method of reminding.

Put up a note on the refrigerator or on the computer at work. Some people are in the habit of sticking note everywhere as reminders. Change the spot and color of the note every week or every other day. If one week it was on the computer, put it on the mirror the next or on the phone. Be creative with your reminders and have fun, taking medication will then be fun too.

Make a personal chart. Use different colored pens or paper for the different medications that have to be taken. This is a very neat and organized method and has been proven to work. If all of the above fails get a relative or friend to call and remind you is a good method though it may not be very effective. It may not be effective because once the person hangs up you might forget again. It is better to take the medication while still on the phone just in case you are extra forgetful.

If you are tech savvy set a reminder on your computer or phone. Have a free service send a reminder e-mail if possible. Instruct the e-mail service to keep sending the e mail until you have finally taken the medication. The e-mail can then be deleted.

Come up with other creative ways you think will work for you. Experiment with a few and stick to one that best helps you remember. Regulate yourself and you will never forget taking your medications again.

FAQs' Pertaining To High BP

As you age, you should start taking charge of your health and get to know your body a bit better? If you monitor your blood pressure then you can prevent certain complex health conditions from taking place, like kidney disease, heart problems and even strokes. This article will serve as a guide to educate you on the subject - blood pressure. Anybody can experience high blood pressure, thus ethnicity, race, age and gender does not matter. Those having high blood pressure are more prone to developing heart diseases like stroke in comparison to individuals with normal blood pressure.

What is meant by high blood pressure? High blood pressure can be defined as the force exerted by the blood on the artery walls. Blood pressure rises and falls on a daily basis in case of a person with regular blood pressure but for individuals with high blood pressure, it rises and ceases, and there is no reduction in the pressure. Any figure lesser than 120 and more than 80 is considered to be a normal blood pressure. Here, 120 s the systolic blood pressure level while 80 is the diastolic blood pressure level. Individuals having a blood pressure will have 140 over 90 or even higher levels.

Systolic blood pressure is described as the force of the blood present in the arteries when the heart is beating. The force of the blood present in the arteries when the heart is in relaxation mode is called diastolic blood pressure.

Are there any risks associated with high blood pressure? There are many risks associated with high blood pressure including heart diseases and strokes. While some of the risks factors of high blood pressure can be modified, others cannot be. Some examples of risk factors would be abnormal level of cholesterol, diabetes, lack of physical activity, tobacco and obesity.

Who is prone to developing high blood pressure? When it comes to any particular segment of population, it is the African Americans who win hands down. About one out of every three American adults suffers from high blood pressure. When compared with white Americans, African Americans experience a substantially higher death rate from stroke and diseases pertaining to the kidney. However, the good news is that blood pressure can be monitored and lowered with the help of the right treatment.

It is quite fortunate that there are umpteen ways of bringing down one's level of blood pressure. Out of these, exercise is a great and foolproof method. If you want to make your heart stronger as you get older then you should start following an exercise regime or routine regularly. Why is it necessary to make the heart stronger? Well, if your heart is strong then it would be able to pump blood more easily and reduce chances of developing kidney diseases or stroke. Thus, one should start exercising from today itself.

It is always a good idea to consult a doctor or general physician if you are worried about your blood pressure as he/she can prescribe medications for you while taking your lifestyle and health into consideration.

www.ingramcontent.com/pod-product-compliance
Lightning Source LLC
Chambersburg PA
CBHW070501290526
45790CB00003B/1052